A real swinish book

Thomas M. Meine

Fat Pig Willi

A salutary lesson
– not only for children

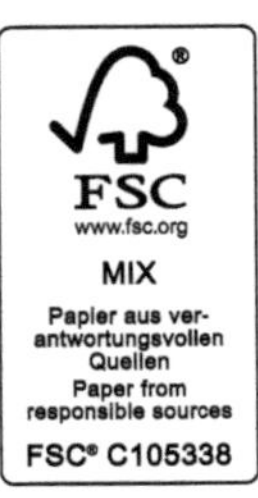

Bibliographic information published by the
Deutsche Nationalbibliothek:

The Deutsche Nationalbibliothek lists this publication in the
Deutsche Nationalbibliografie; detailed bibliographic data
are available on the Internet at http://dnb.dnb.de

© 2025 Thomas M. Meine
Publisher: BoD · Books on Demand GmbH,
Überseering 33, 22297 Hamburg, bod@bod.de
Print: Libri Plureos GmbH, Friedensallee 273,
22763 Hamburg

2nd edition June 2025

ISBN: 978-3-7568-0933-2

The piggish content:

Page

I. On a farm

On a small farm, somewhere in the countryside, a farmer, his wife, their two children, and the animals lived happily together.

I can't remember exactly where it was, but I will never forget the exciting story of Fat Pig Willi.

Willi is a boar, as male pigs are called, but that is not so important. The problem began because Willi ate everything he could find and didn't exercise at all. So, it's no surprise that he was getting fatter and fatter every day.

He slept in the stable with a chicken, a goat, and a sheep. Sometimes, the cat and dog would also come inside to find a nice spot to rest.

And I shall not forget Spike, a big rooster. He woke up everyone in the morning with his loud crowing. He did this every day and as early as he could, because the earlier he raised his voice, the more important he felt.

All the animals, except for Willi, ran around the estate during the day. When the weather was nice, they stayed outside as long as possible and only came back to the barn when it was time to eat.

Willi was very lazy. He liked to stay inside and only moved when the grub was put in his trough, but then he was always first. He pushed the other animals out of the way, stepped on their food, and quickly emptied his trough, making loud noises. He always looked to see if he could take food from the others. After eating, he lay down again and fell asleep, snoring.

Even though all pigs enjoy rolling in the dirt, Willi didn't care much for it. He thought the way back was just too far. He only went to the muddy puddle to roll on his back a couple of times when his skin itched. He was too lazy to return to the stable for his nap, so he often fell asleep right on the spot.

But mostly, Willi stayed in the stable and slept all day in his favourite corner. Using his big nose, he moved straw and litter from the other animals' spots to his, making it softer and more comfortable.

Willy grew fatter and fatter because he never stopped eating and didn't like to move. He also became lazier as he gained weight, and the lazier he became, the more weight he gained.

Willi soon found it hard to walk, but he didn't mind because exercise wasn't his thing anyway.

However, his big belly soon became a larger problem: It was dragging on the ground. This caused him pain and made it harder to move, and the less he moved, the bigger his belly got, causing even more pain, further reducing his desire to move.

After a while, he stopped going to his favourite spot and fell asleep next to the trough after wolfing his food and that of some of his friends.

The other animals always warned him, 'Willi, stop eating so much, and move around more, or this will end badly', but Willi never listened to them.

II. Cleaning the stable

Even though the stable was cleaned every day, it sometimes needed a more intense washdown. In this case, everything inside had to be taken out beforehand.

First, the animals were sent outside. Then, the farmer and his wife pulled everything not firmly attached to the ground through the stable door and into the open.

After that, all the dirt followed. The floor was sprayed with a strong stream of water, and the murky broth was pushed outside with a big broom.

But this time, they had a major problem before coming to the final step: Everyone was outside except Willi, who was still sleeping in his corner.

»Come on, Willi!« yelled the farmer, but Willi just gave him a sidelong glance and then fell asleep again.

»Leave him alone!« the farmer's wife said. »Let's give him his rest as long as we have everything else outside!«

But finally, it was Willi's turn.

»Can't we clean around him first?« asked the farmer's wife. »Then we can roll him to the side and clean underneath«, she added.

»Are you crazy?« said the farmer. Willi has to go outside like everyone else!«

Willi, still half asleep, heard it. 'If there is no other choice', he thought, 'I might as well go outside too'. So he got up slowly and walked to the door, dragging along some dirt from the stable that stuck to his belly.

III. What a mess!

When Willi got to the stable door, he stopped for a moment to let his eyes adjust to the bright sunlight.

The weather was nice; the sun was shining, it was warm, and a light breeze made the air feel fresh.

The other animals were already playing and having fun outside.

Willi wanted to go slowly outside, but then something bad happened – something terribly bad: He got stuck in the door.

He pushed with all his might, first forward and then backwards, and forward and backwards, but he couldn't move at all.

Willi was trapped, and his big, fat body was pressed against the door frame.

»Come on, Willi!« shouted the farmer, but Willi couldn't move an inch, neither forwards nor backwards; it was all in vain.

The rooster was the first to see what was going on and jumped down from the dungheap.

He went over, looked at the problem, and commented like a 'real expert:

»Willi is stuck; he can't get out anymore.«

The farmer in the stable had also seen what was wrong. He went to the door and pushed Willi from behind, but it didn't work, no matter how hard he tried.

Finally, he lost his balance and fell headfirst into the dirt.

»What a piggish mess!« he yelled.

IV. What now?

The goat thought this was very funny and showed his feelings by an excited bleating, whereupon the sheep gave a stern look at the goat and said:

»No time for fun! The stable must be cleaned, and Willi needs to get out the door first!«

The farmer's wife came to help her husband, and both tried hard to push Willi out.

»Together! Together!« shouted the farmer at his wife. »We must push together!« It didn't help. Willi stayed right where he was.

Meanwhile, all the animals gathered at the door while the farmer and his wife were locked in the stable behind Willi.

Willi heard the voices around him, sometimes yelling around, and sometimes addressing him directly.

Soon, it became so noisy that no one could understand a word anymore.

They gave all sorts of advice and comfort, but were also upset because the day's plans had been interrupted by Willy.

Everyone was convinced: 'He should have exercised more and eaten less. We've told him that many times!«

The chicken contributed to the chaos in their special way:

First, each hen gave her own opinion, and then, when they all agreed, they clucked together until one of them had a new idea, and the confusion started all over again.

Meanwhile, Willi stood pinched in the doorway, looking very sad.

»Yes«, he said, »you were right. I should have moved around a little more.« But he didn't say anything about eating less; that was probably too hard for him to admit, even in this bad situation.

After lengthy discussions, more useful advice was given:

»The door frame needs to be removed!« said one of them.

We should leave him there without food for a few days«, said another …

… and the sheep suggested: »Maybe we can put some grease on the door beams to make them slippery?«

And then others wanted to try again by using force:

»It might work if they push from the back inside while someone pulls from the front.«

In the meantime, the farmers' two children came home. Tristan, the older one, immediately got a rope and tied it around Willi's fat neck.

His younger sister Irene joined him at the end of the rope to help him pull.

While their parents pushed and pushed, as hard as they could, the kids pulled and pulled until Willi couldn't breathe anymore.

It did not work. Willi was stuck even tighter than before, and the fat bulges on his sides were now clawing right and left around the door frame like thick fingers.

V. A sparkling idea

Finally, the rooster had an idea: »Move aside!« he said and jumped onto Willi's back.

»Move aside, both of you!« he crowed again as he looked with a scowl at the farmer and his wife.

He fluttered off Willi's back, went past the farmer couple, and took a position at the very end of the stable.

»Does he want to sit there in the shade and watch from inside?« asked the sheep, and everyone was eager to see what would happen next.

The bigger animals moved closer to Willi to look over him, and the chickens flew up into the air. They all wanted to see what was happening inside.

The rooster straightened up and puffed out his chest. He had his eyes firmly fixed on Willi, and his feet scratched nervously on the floor.

While they all watched in suspense, he suddenly ran forward.

The farmer's wife threw her hands up into the air and said, »I hope he doesn't want to shove Willi with a running start! He's just going to bang his head.«

The rooster's long, thin legs moved faster and faster, supported by a powerful flapping of his wings.

Everyone was amazed and held their breath. They had never seen a rooster run so fast. No one knew what he was up to, but that would soon become clear ...

VI. Great panic in the countryside

Suddenly, the animals and the children eagerly waiting in front of Willi jumped chaotically to the side and fell over each other in great panic.

The chickens scattered apart in all directions so violently that their feathers flew around through the air as if Mother Holle would shake out her beds.

But what made everyone so scared?

At full speed and still a few feet away from Willi, the rooster had raised his head. His eyes sparkled like lightning, and the long, sharp beak was now pointing forward like a knight's lance, ready to strike.

The sheep had landed beside the goat.

The kids were piled on top of each other.

The dog and cat howled in such a horrible way that you couldn't tell who was who.

The chickens were still in the air when fat Willi slipped out below them.

A horrible squeal filled their ears: Willi had been hit at full speed in the butt by the rooster's beak.

The door was shaking – no, the whole stable was shaking – as Willi slipped out.

Because of his big belly, his feet barely had contact with the ground, and he shovelled around like crazy.

Like a police car turning up the siren and going around in circles in the garden, Willi made loud wailing noises, taking one spin after another in panic and pain.

VII. Lucky Willi, that was close!

Willi couldn't sit down anymore. But lying down was also not such a good idea, because when getting up, he had to take an interim position on his butt … Ouch!

He had already been outside for three days on a special diet before he tried to go back into the stable.

But no chance – it took him full three weeks on a strict diet to get back to his quarters.

Even then, he had a hard time getting through the door, and for many days before, he stood shivering in the rain, pressing himself against the stable wall to stay warm.

VIII. A lesson for all

A lot of time has gone by. Willi is eating much less and is not gulping his food. Above all, he moves around a lot more and likes being outside in the fresh air.

The children of the farmers now avoid certain sweets and other 'fatteners'. They help at home when requested and complete their homework without any prompting.

They like to play outside whenever possible, rather than lying around or sitting on the couch.

At school, they shared that story with their classmates, and it had a beneficial effect on the other children.

So, everyone was taking home something good from Willi's story.

IX. The hero

And what about that rooster? Well, he is more adored by the chickens than ever.

You can see his 'Eggselency' sitting at the top of the dungheap, which the farmer made a bit higher for him to show thanks. He proudly puffs up his chest and crows even louder and more self-assured. His louder crow is not the only thing that annoys everyone lately, especially Willi – Spike now starts crowing five minutes earlier than he usually does.

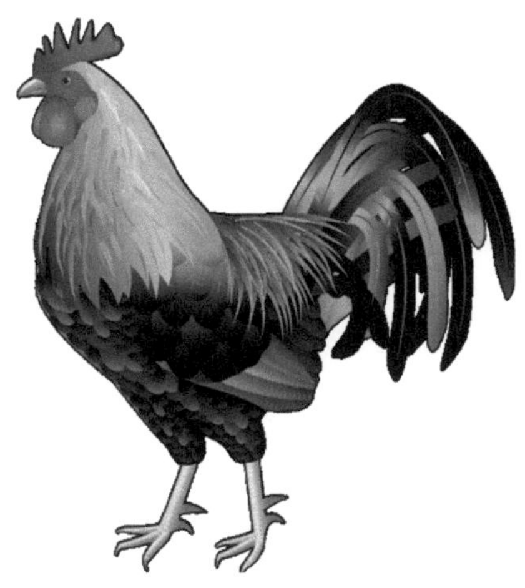